Botched Girl Summer!

The Unofficial Guide for International Plastic Surgery & Cosmetic Dentistry

Erika Sato, MD
&
Andre Jordan, DDS

Copyright © 2021
All rights reserved. No part of this book may be reproduced, scanned, or distributed in any printed or electronic form without permission.
First Edition: July 2021
Edited by Uzo Odili, MD
Published by The Book Patch, LLC – http://thebp.site/308063
Printed in the United States of America

BOTCHED GIRL SUMMER!

THE UNOFFICIAL GUIDE FOR INTERNATIONAL PLASTIC SURGERY & COSMETIC DENTISTRY

Botched Girl Summer! The Unofficial Travel Guide

TABLE OF CONTENTS

Heart to Heart with Dr. Erika Sato 1

The Whole TRUTH with Dr. Andre Jordan 4

To Fly or Not to Fly 8

Plastic Surgery 101 12

How to Not Die if you go International 22

Spirit Airlines Now Boarding to Colombia 27

Costa Rica - Pura Vida! 33

Bienvenidos à Mexico! 38

Phuket! Let's Go to Thailand! 42

Final Thoughts 46

Erika Sato, MD & Andre Jordan, DDS

Disclaimer – Although this book contains information about detailed plastic surgery and cosmetic dentistry procedures, this guide is not a substitute for a medical consultation. Please consult with your physician for a detailed assessment of your surgical needs and the procedures that would best satisfy them.

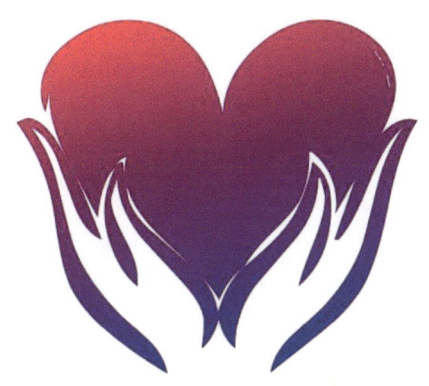

Heart to Heart with Dr. Erika Sato

My name is Erika Sato, MD. I'm a double board-certified Plastic Surgeon, and I love my job. I am honored to have the privilege of meeting wonderful people every day and helping their vision of a beautiful self-image become reality. I currently practice in Houston, Texas at My Houston Surgeons, and I have openings for new consultations every week.

Traveling for plastic surgery and cosmetic dentistry has increased in volume year over year for over a decade. We see the trend and we think it's going in the wrong direction. Modern medicine has improved safety of surgical procedures and improved the beauty of the finished product. Unfortunately, most countries don't offer the same level of infrastructure and basic standards to produce an equivalent quality of surgical care. There are a few exceptions, but it is nearly impossible to know where it is safe and where it isn't unless you are an expert in the field. This book was designed to educate potential patients and guide them through the process of selecting a surgeon that will increase chances of a successful surgical experience. We know that you want the best boob job and butt lift for your money, but we also know that you want to wake up after surgery and come home safely to your family.

We get it. We understand that modifying your body is a delicate subject. You care about your self-image, but you also care about getting the body you want at a price you can afford. We want you to have the body of your dreams in the safest and most affordable way possible. Nobody wants to think about what might happen if plastic surgery goes wrong. But complications can happen with surgery, and if they do happen to you, you want to be in a country with excellent medical care in every category, not just plastic surgery. My goal is to educate patients, so that they can make an informed decision when deciding whether to stay local or travel out of the country for cosmetic plastic surgery.

You might compare prices in the United States to prices in another country and decide that saving $5000 is worth the risk of leaving the U.S. for your cosmetic makeover. It's true that we take a risk multiple times a day and survive unscathed. When we get behind the wheel of a car, there is a risk of having an automobile accident. When we fly on an airplane, there is a risk of a plane crash. These risks exist and they don't keep everyone from driving or flying. Approximately 1 in 8 women will develop breast cancer and we don't advise that all women routinely get prophylactic mastectomies. I totally understand that some patients have the mindset that they will still travel for the better price. If someone offered you the Maserati or Ferrari of your dreams for $5000 less than the regular price, you would be crazy not to at least consider the option. Just remember that plastic surgery is still real surgery. The outcomes of the procedures may be more playful or sexy, but the risks are real. The rate of complications in plastic surgery ranges from 0.1% to 50%. The risk varies because there are very good plastic surgeons all over the world, but there are also health factors that cannot be controlled. I honestly believe all major travel destinations for plastic surgery have at least a few very good plastic surgeons, but usually they are not more affordable than a comparable option here in the United States.

The average cost to see a Plastic Surgeon here in the U.S. for a complication, knowing that a different surgeon performed your procedure, is $350 for the consultation. The cost skyrockets if the patient needs any treatment procedures, like drainage of fluid or a surgical revision. There's no guarantee that medical insurance plans will cover the care related to these complications. People call almost every day to ask about an appointment to evaluate their overseas complications, but they don't book the appointment when they find out that a consultation for fixing complications isn't free. The people who travel overseas to save money on up-front costs are likely the same people who don't want to pay or can't afford to pay for necessary post-op care here in the U.S.

If you have researched the risks and you still plan to travel abroad for your medical procedure, this book provides a checklist to help guide you through your journey successfully. We have asked the important questions for each of the top countries for Medical Tourism.

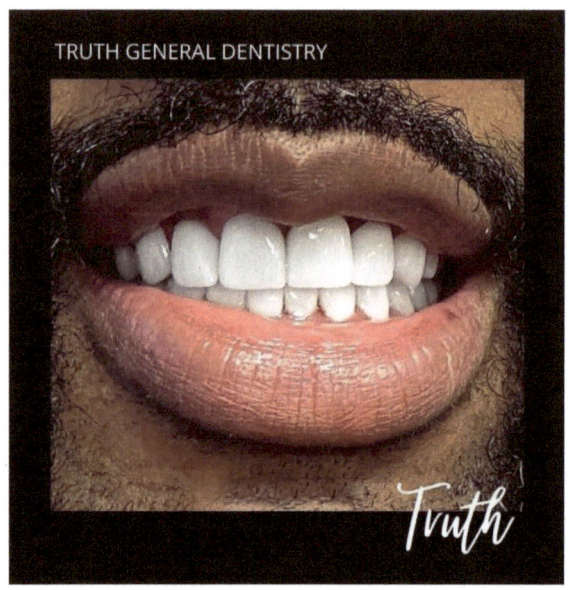

THE WHOLE TRUTH WITH DR. ANDRE JORDAN

"Do you do veneers?" Inevitability, that is the question people often ask me that leads into the conversation of dental tourism. My name is Dr. Andre Jordan, Doctor of Dental Surgery and founder of Truth General Dentistry in Houston, TX. When I first started my path in dentistry, I never really pictured myself advertising as a Cosmetic Dentist. One thing that I quickly realized with regards to dentistry is that your style of dentistry will find you organically. After practicing dentistry for 10 years now, my reputation has attracted patients interested in cosmetic dentistry. As such, cosmetics has become a very large portion of the total scope of my dental practice. I am also a self-professed world traveler and commercial aviation enthusiast. This blend of hobby and career has put me in the direct path of dental tourism.

Just like medical tourism, dental tourism is the practice of traveling outside of the United States to seek dental work. The allure of traveling to a foreign, exotic land to seek out the world's foremost expert in the world's foremost field of study has an element of seductiveness. In reality, it's quite the opposite. The bulk of the population that seeks dental or medical work outside of the U.S. are doing so in search of a deal ... not better treatment or higher quality care ... only a cheaper price. The would-be savings hunters may disguise that key part of the conversation in various ways, but it is only to dress up the reality that they are going because it is cheaper.

If you are considering becoming a dental/medical tourist or you already have your bags packed, your assumption might be that I would be vehemently against it because I'm an American dentist. Not necessarily ... the reality is, patients that are gung-ho about dental/medical tourism oftentimes make very poor clients as we will address as well. Dental/Medical work performed outside of the United States would be legitimately cheaper in other countries if those countries have a favorable exchange rate. Material Costs, Dental Education Costs, and Labor Costs should only be compared and calculated against the exchange rate if the quality of work and safety standards are even. It's quite possible that with some economic relationships, the savings costs may not justify the costs of travel or hiccups that may occur. When the comparison numbers are favorable towards saving money with travel, the old adage, "If it sounds too good to be true, then it probably is" is scarily accurate. At some of the prices that some clinicians are charging outside of the U.S. – it is IMPOSSIBLE for the work to be of the same caliber and offer the same protection against personal liability. At certain price points, the quality of materials, cleanliness of materials, regulations regarding dental protocols, training level of clinicians, and your personal safety must be questioned.

To establish a baseline for comparison, let's talk about the United States of America. Dentists and Medical Doctors in America are often labeled as being greedy and money hungry. Some people believe that the high cost of dental and medical care in the United States is unfairly marked up for personal gain. The United States healthcare system is far from perfect, and I cannot attest that the pursuit of profits doesn't drive the industry. Nor do I think Doctors should be apologetic for earning a very good living from their craft; especially if it is earned ethically. In the United States, Medical and Dental school programs are highly competitive; oftentimes an incoming medical or dental school class may consist of 50 to 200 students at most in each respective school – with an application pool in the thousands.

After a high school diploma is obtained, a 4-year college degree in a curriculum that contains medical or dental prerequisites must also be obtained. Technically, if you demonstrate a masterful comprehension of the undergraduate course content, proven by a strong academic record – you can apply to Medical or Dental school prior to finishing an undergraduate program. Of course, a strong academic record and good scores on the Medical College Admission Test (MCAT) or Dental Admission Test (DAT) are required to get an in-person interview.

Medical and Dental school are a subsequent 4 years after the undergraduate level, and a dental school or medical school education – not including an undergraduate degree can cost as much as $500,000. After a demonstration of proficiency in the respective training programs, competency is verified by several standardized national board exams and state licensure exams. In most cases post-graduate residency programs would be required before practicing the selected field of practice...which imparts another level of competition and costs. The length of those post-graduate programs after the high school/college/med-dent school gauntlet ranges from one year to 8 years. Therefore, the realistic minimum amount of education that your dentist may have before treating you after high school is 8 years. Meanwhile your Medical Doctor may have a minimum of 12+ years. That alone is enough to justify the cost of healthcare in America.

If we look at the business of healthcare in America – it boils down to cost of manufacturing and labor costs. America has a minimum wage. Those factors above establish the baseline of costs before we even begin to talk about profit margins. We also have not addressed the inherent medicolegal liability that exists and cost to insure against lawsuits due to the fact that healthcare providers are working with what was divinely created...the human body is not a toaster. My official stance and purpose of this book is to arm those on the fence with dos and don'ts so that you don't get injured or killed in the process.

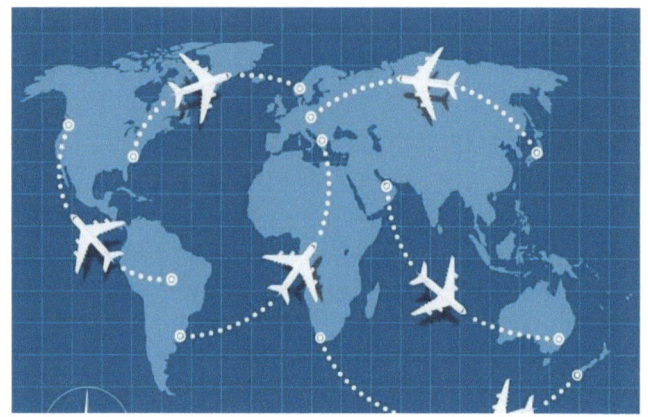

To Fly or Not to Fly
-Erika Sato, MD

Whether you want to explore the Central American rainforests while you search for a surgeon, relax on the beach recovering from your mommy makeover, or you want to relax oceanside after you complete your veneers, the world offers a variety of beautiful options for travel medicine. You know by now that it is much more affordable to have plastic surgery outside of the U.S. in places like Columbia, Dominican Republic, and Mexico. This more affordable cost allows patients who otherwise couldn't afford the surgery or justify the spend, a more cost-effective option. It also entices patients who desire multiple procedures to be done at one time but can only afford to do one procedure if done here in the U.S. However, having a lower up-front cost doesn't mean that the total cost will be lower. Just like buying a cash car that costs less up front, there's a very real possibility that the car will break down and cost you much more in the future.

The up-front cost of surgery is less, what about the cost of flight, hotel, and your companion. Most procedures are so extensive that you will require another adult present to assist you with activities of daily life and any dressing changes that are needed. What about your childcare while you are gone? Other countries are not necessarily cheaper than Miami – it's cheap because they don't have a medical office where they do pre- and post-op care. It's like shopping on Amazon because it's easier and faster, when you really need to go into Best Buy and do a thorough evaluation of the options, not just look at pictures. Because the doctor doesn't need to pay rent for an office, they can offer you a lower price, but they also don't offer any follow up visits. They might not even have a phone number to call back. Even if the staff does answer the phone, they might tell you the doctor is out and never call you back.

If you travel for a procedure and then try to follow up with a doctor here in the U.S., be prepared to spend more money. Medical insurance doesn't usually pay for treatment of complications of cosmetic plastic surgery. Plastic surgeons here do not give free follow-up after a procedure that another surgeon performed.

Another reason people travel for plastic surgery is related to the lack of regulation on procedures overseas. In many countries, there is no regulation on how long the patient can be under anesthesia or how much lipoaspirate can be taken out. Overseas, plastic surgeons can keep you under general anesthesia for as long as they want – 12 hours or longer. It means a lot of procedures can be combined at one time, which appeals to patients despite the increased risk.

Here in the U.S., we have guidelines and regulations that recommend limits on procedure time (time under general anesthesia) and fat removal volume (total lipoaspirate). These regulations help keep you safe by preventing procedures from becoming too risky. They vary from state to state. In Texas, the safe amount of lipoaspirate is 5 liters (lipoaspirate = fat mixed with blood, interstitial fluid, and tumescent fluid). If you have more than 5 liters removed (or 4 liters in Florida), you are supposed to stay overnight in a medical facility with continued monitoring and a nurse at your bedside, usually with IV fluids running and a foley catheter to drain your bladder.

The recommended maximum time under general anesthesia is 6.5h-7h. The safety guidelines also recommend that a surgeon who performs a procedure that lasts 7h or longer should keep the patient overnight in a hospital or equivalent monitoring facility overnight for safety. The overnight stay adds cost for the patient, as much as $1500 for the night if done at a surgery center and more if at a large hospital. Surgeons in other countries do not have to abide by these guidelines so they will offer you longer anesthesia times, more combined procedures, and higher fat volumes removed in one-day procedures and send you back to the hotel or non-medical recovery suite that night.

If you have undergone previous plastic surgery, a c-section delivery, or any other major surgery in the past, you probably know that you need to have assistance with the activities of daily living immediately after the surgery. Nice hotels offer excellent room service, but they don't offer bedside nursing care. If you travel for surgery without a helper, you may have a much more difficult time during your recovery at the hotel.

Another potential difference you want to know is that the sterilization standards in other countries are not the same as the U.S. The training for plastic surgeons is not as long or as rigorous in many countries. There is no medical malpractice insurance, so no one to quickly settle a lawsuit if you sue when something goes wrong. And let's be real ... that "something" could be death. For the Brazilian Butt Lift, the rate of death is 7% when you have your surgery out of the country, compared to the U.S., where it's 1/11,500 (safer than a cholecystectomy) and in Miami a little higher at 1/10,000. Of course, it's not zero risk, but 1 death out of 11,500 patients is much safer than 7 deaths out of 100.

Another question to consider is where will you be recovering? Will you recover after surgery in a standard post-anesthesia care unit in a proper medical facility or at a "recovery house" with non-medical care takers? A good nurse will prevent complications after surgery and there's no substitute for that.

If you develop a complication out of the country, what is your plan? Will you stay long enough to take care of it? Does your insurance (if you have health insurance) work there? The window for the big complications is 2 weeks. Are you planning on staying that long? Once you stay for 2 weeks is the cost still lower? You are at increased risk for a deep vein thrombosis (DVT) or pulmonary embolism (PE) if you fly within 2 weeks of your surgery. So, if you leave before you are 2 weeks out from surgery, you are putting yourself at increased risk of a PE (this can kill you) if you take a flight.

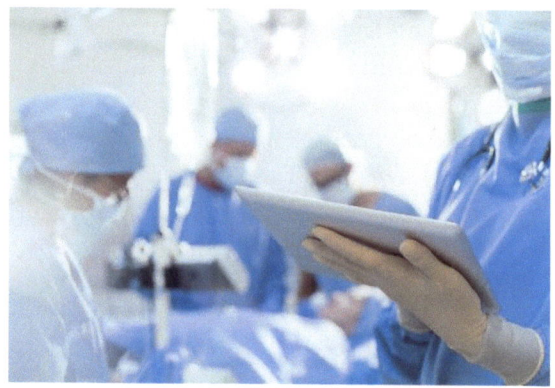

PLASTIC SURGERY 101
-ERIKA SATO, MD

Breast Augmentation (BAM)

Breasts are often the first thing a person notices after walking into a room. When you consider augmenting such an important part of your image, you have to make sure that you take every safety precaution possible. There are some specific questions you need to think about before you choose another country for your breast augmentation. Are the implants you receive in this other country FDA approved? It is not uncommon for plastic surgeons in the U.S. to remove implants that literally have no labeling. Breast implants that are manufactured under appropriate regulations have information engraved onto them. Off-brand and illegal breast implants don't have any of that. Can you tell the difference? If you look at it, you can't read any important info like size, manufacturer, or contents. This is scary because you do not know the sterility or integrity of the implant that is inside of your body.

Breast augmentation is one of the most popular plastic surgery procedures in the United States. Breast augmentation can give women a more proportionate figure and help them to feel more confident about their appearance. Breast implants are silicone shells filled with either saline (salt water) or silicone gel. Both silicone breast implants and saline implants are safe, and each offers its own advantages. Gummy bear implants are a newer type of silicone implant and are quite popular because of the advantages they offer over traditional silicone implants. They are also known as form-stable implants. When gummy bear implants experience a rupture, they maintain their shape quite well, and there is no leaking of the material, because they are filled with a denser or more cohesive gel.

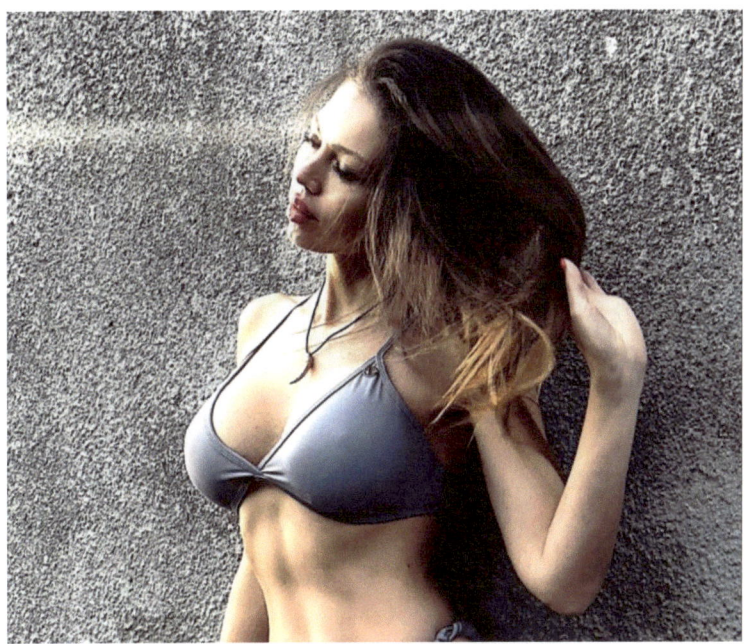

Breast augmentations have their own possible complications, and the risk increases if the BAM is done in conjunction with a breast lift, which adds more skin excision and movement of the nipple-areola complex (NAC).

Infection – If an infection occurs around a foreign body such as a breast implant it can be very difficult or impossible to treat with antibiotics as the infection can seed the implant. Just like how insects dig underground to avoid predators and pesticides, bacteria can permeate the plastic implant, living just out of reach of antibiotic treatment. In many cases, the implant will have to be removed. A new one cannot be placed until at least 6 weeks later to ensure that the infection has been treated appropriately before putting the new implant into the same space. The cost of the surgery to remove the implant along with the cost of the future surgery to place a new implant (including the cost of the new implant) is the responsibility of the patient. Infection can occur in the U.S., but our sterility guidelines and laws are very strict compared to other countries, so our risk is lower.

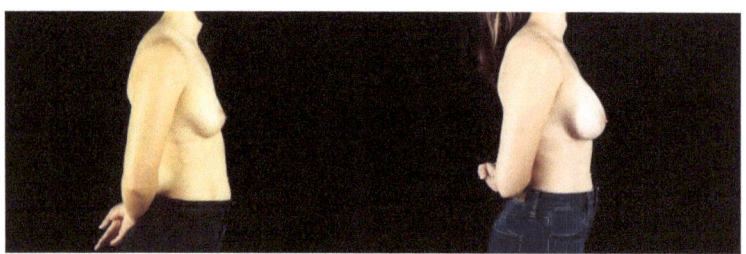

Bleeding or hematoma – if the patient has significant bleeding post op blood can collect in the space around the implant. This will lead to risk for infection if left. The patient is usually taken back to the OR asap to wash the pocket out and salvage the implant. Bleeding post op occurs usually because the patient's blood pressure is low while under anesthesia then once they are awake and can feel pain/anxiety their blood pressure increases leading to bleeding that wasn't present in the surgery.

Capsular contracture – 7-15% of patients will develop this in the lifetime of the implant (average lifetime is 10 years) at no fault to the surgeon or the patient. This is when the body somewhat "rejects" the implant and builds scar tissue circumferentially around the implant to wall it off from the body. The breast implant companies will provide a replacement implant here in the U.S. if this occurs within a specific time frame. Is this the case in the country they are considering traveling to for their surgery?

Consider your general follow up needs after surgery. What if you aren't sure if you are having a complication or if what you are experiencing is "normal". You just want the surgeon to see you and make sure everything is okay. Will you travel back for this and incur those costs? Most plastic surgeons here in the U.S. charge $350 per visit to see a patient they did not operate on for follow up. They then charge more to treat any complication if one is found. This can add up to a lot of money in a hurry. Alternatively, if you have your surgery here, follow up costs for a defined amount of time is included in the upfront payment (~6 months to one year).

If the BAM is combined with a breast lift or the breast lift is done without an implant, you risk wound breakdown with possible exposure of the implant, skin necrosis with possible exposure of the implant, and partial or full NAC loss from ischemia. The larger the implant that is used in conjunction with the breast lift, the higher the risk of the above complications. Serious complications need ongoing wound care or another surgery to debride the dead tissue and reconstruct the breast. This may take months to heal.

Brazilian Butt Lift (BBL)

Butt augmentation procedures work to reshape and enhance the buttocks to create a rounder, smoother and more shapely appearance. With the popularity of curvaceous celebrities like Kim Kardashian and Beyonce, many people are looking to achieve that coveted hourglass figure. There are different ways to achieve these goals such as high-volume fat grafting ("Brazilian butt lift"), buttock implants, or skin tightening (traditional buttock lift). Butt augmentation procedures can be combined and are tailored to the needs of each patient.

Implant-based butt augmentation involves incisions made near the gluteal cleft or in the lower buttock crease followed by insertion of synthetic buttock implants to create generous curves. This procedure is performed under general anesthesia and is mostly recommended for patients who have flat backsides and limited fatty tissue elsewhere on the body. Buttock implants which are made of soft silicone are inserted into the gluteal muscle or in the folds between the cheeks right above the pelvic bone for a lifted and shapelier figure.

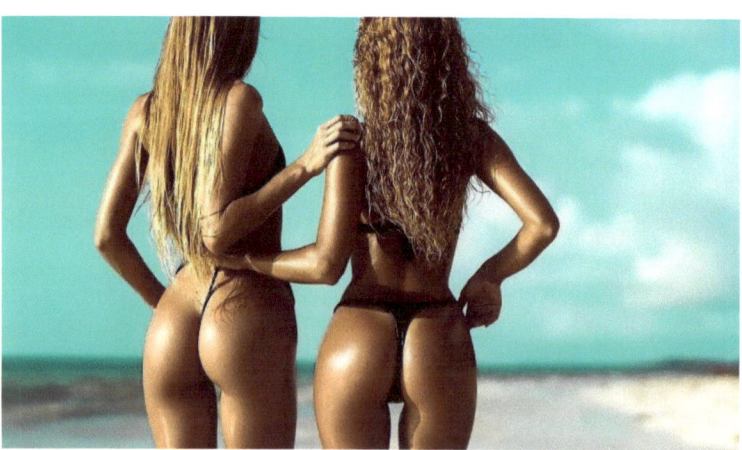

A traditional butt augmentation more commonly known as a "buttock lift" or "posterior body lift" is performed by creating an incision across the lower back, where hanging skin is lifted, trimmed, and then sutured. Liposuction can also be performed in adjacent areas for complete gluteal contouring and fat grafting.

To achieve your desired body profile, a "Brazilian butt lift" can create a shapelier, more filled out and lifted backside. The way a Brazilian butt lift works is by using your own fat (autologous fat transfer) to augment the gluteal area or buttocks and/or hips. Fat is harvested through liposuction, processed until purified, and then injected into the buttocks and/or hips for a natural enhancement. With a Brazilian butt lift, the typical areas that are liposuctioned to harvest fat are the abdomen, waistline, back, and love handles. To achieve more volume, liposuction can also be performed on other areas of the body such as the thighs and arms in order to collect more fat for injection.

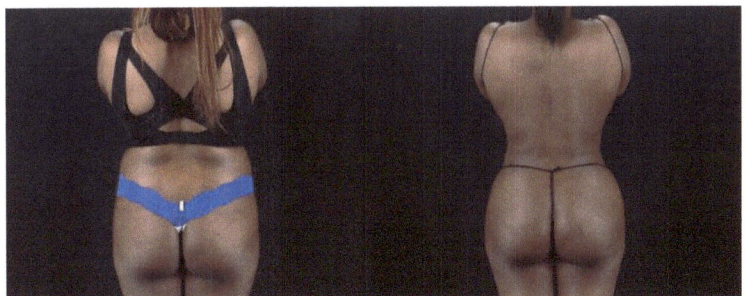

Patients who are unhappy with the shape and appearance of their buttocks and have good donor fat are considered the best candidates for a Brazilian butt lift. This is an outpatient procedure which is performed under general anesthesia. The areas around the buttocks are sculpted to make the augmentation more pronounced.

After a Brazilian butt lift, you will not be able to apply direct pressure such as sitting or lying on the buttocks for about 10 days. For several weeks, you will wear a tight compression garment with molded buttocks to help shape and apply uniform pressure to the areas of liposuction. You will not take the compression garment off for extended periods of time during the first 3-5 days post op but will undo the garment daily to do "skin checks" as the garment can be abrasive and may cause the skin to tear. The garment will be worn for 4-6 weeks total and must remain tight, or a smaller size must be purchased. After the 2nd week post-surgery as the swelling starts to subside, most patients require a smaller size garment. Lipo foam and lipo boards along with baby powder and pads can be applied under your garment to protect your skin.

At your first postoperative visit at 2-5 days after your BBL surgery, Dr. Sato will take the compression garment off. At this point you will be able to go home and shower. You must wear a compression garment (to control swelling) ~23 hours per day for 4-6 weeks except when taking a shower or washing the garment. There may be intermittent swelling in the areas of liposuction for up to 6 months. You should be able to resume all normal activities at 4-6 weeks post op (varies from patient to patient depending on how active your lifestyle is). Fat volume loss can occur up to 3 months after your surgery.

Another option for patients who are thin and do not have enough fat for a Brazilian butt lift is to increase the size of the buttocks using Sculptra, a poly-L-lactic acid that plumps by stimulating your body's own collagen production.

Abdominoplasty (Tummy Tuck)

Abdominoplasty, commonly known as a tummy tuck, is a surgical procedure used to flatten and shape the abdomen by removing excess skin and fat and tightening the muscles of the abdominal wall. A tummy tuck is an ideal procedure for women who have pockets of fat and loose skin that have not responded to traditional reduction efforts like diet and exercise. Abdominoplasty is frequently performed on women after pregnancy with striae (stretch marks) and excess skin, and on men and women after significant weight loss from diet, exercise, or surgery. For this reason, it is often a procedure done as part of post-bariatric surgery or a mommy makeover.

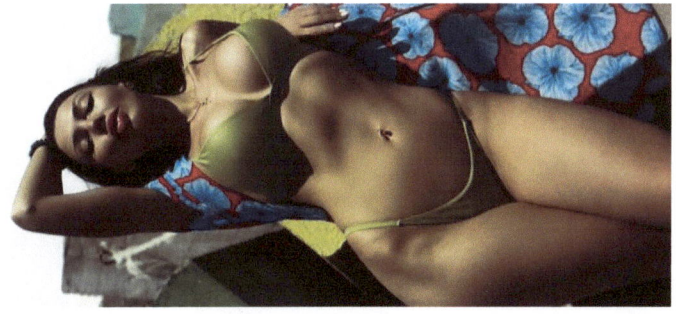

A tummy tuck is usually an outpatient procedure done under local anesthetic and IV sedation at our in-office operating room or under general anesthesia at an ambulatory surgery center. The procedure is highly customized based on your needs, so the length of surgery can vary greatly. For a full abdominoplasty, Dr. Sato will make an incision from one hip bone to the other, low along the pubic hair line. She will remove the excess skin, tighten and repair the abdominal muscles, and reshape the abdominal silhouette. Liposuction will be used to remove excess fat, and the navel is retained in its proper location.

After the surgery, your abdomen will be bandaged, and a compression garment will be worn to help reduce swelling. You will experience some soreness, bruising, and swelling. If subcutaneous drains were placed intra-operatively, you will be provided with drain teaching. Most people take 10 days to 2 weeks off from work for their recovery. Heavy lifting (> 10 lbs) and strenuous activity are discouraged for 4-6 weeks. Dr. Sato will give you full instructions for post-operative care and will monitor your progress during follow-up visits. There will be some scarring from either full or partial abdominoplasty, but these will fade significantly over time and can usually be hidden under clothing including swimwear and lingerie.

The price of an abdominoplasty is impacted by many factors. The length of the procedure, the particulars of the surgical technique, and the amount of tissue removed all play a role in determining the cost of a tummy tuck.

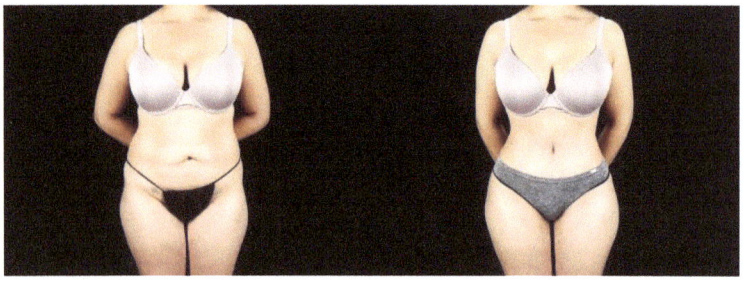

What are the risks involved with having a tummy tuck here or internationally? The separation of the skin and fat layers from the abdominal wall creates the potential for free fluid to fill the space in between. When free fluid collects in between these layers, that complication is called a seroma.

Seromas can be detected early during the second week after surgery. Initial treatment begins with using a large gauge needle and syringe to aspirate, or suck out, the seroma fluid once or twice a week with a compression dressing. Smaller seromas will resolve after five or six aspirations and a few weeks of compression. Without routine follow up to ensure that seromas heal, the problem will get worse. Larger seromas can require additional treatment such as application of irritants to the inner surface to stimulate the two surfaces to scar together. If those measures fail, the surgery may have to be revised.

Deep vein thrombosis is another complication that commonly occurs after surgery. Whether you sit still on a long flight or lie flat on the surgery table, if you don't move your legs for several hours, your blood doesn't flow well. When the blood flow of the legs is compromised, a clot can form in the deep veins of your legs. This is caused a deep vein thrombosis (DVT). If the blood clot dislodges and begins to move, it can travel to the lungs and cause a more serious complication called a pulmonary embolus (PE). Both of these medical problems are potentially life-threatening emergencies, but the risk of developing them can be reduced with proper pre-procedural measures and standards of care. Adding the risk of lying flat during a long surgery to the risk of flying overseas after that long surgery, and that's a recipe for potential disaster.

Postoperative pain is both a complication and a normal part of recovery from surgery. Full healing after surgery takes six months or more, as the healing process of muscle is complex. Routine follow up with your surgeon helps patients set reasonable expectations about the pain to come and how best to handle it.

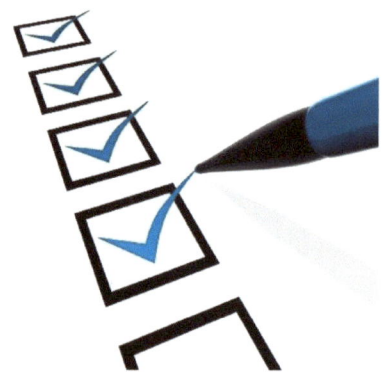

How to Not Die if you go International
-Erika Sato, MD

The DR is not Vegas. What happens overseas does not stay overseas. Even if your surgery seems like it went well in the few days after surgery, it's possible that complications will arise after you return to the U.S. We want you to be aware of the real risks. We know that some of you will still choose to fly overseas for your procedure and that's okay. Take the information that we give you and please use it to stay as safe as possible. Here are the questions you need answered before you book that flight and pay that deposit, no matter what country you choose.

International Travel Medical & Dental Cheat Sheet

☐ Is the surgeon board-certified or properly trained in the field of interest?

☐ What type of training does the country mandate before a doctor can become that type of specialist?
☐ Is the training their surgeon went through comparable to the training here in the U.S.?
☐ Does the country have safe drinking water?
☐ Are procedures regulated for safety in that country?
☐ What is the typical level of cleanliness and sterilization for surgical procedures in that country?
☐ What is the likelihood of a post-surgical infection?
☐ Where will the patient go and be treated should a complication occur?
☐ What is the average level of hospital availability and adequacy of nursing care for post-surgical care?
☐ How will post surgery follow up be handled?
☐ How many times will a patient be seen during that time?
☐ What if a complication occurs after patients return to the U.S.? Will they have any way to speak to their surgeon? Virtual follow up? Or just office staff with the recommendation to travel back to be seen?

After you properly research your destination, you still have to ask yourself some important questions. After you reflect on this checklist, you will know for sure if you are ready to take the plunge into international travel for cosmetic surgery or dentistry.

☐ Does your medical insurance cover the medical stay if anything should go wrong?
☐ Do you want to pay the cost of a medical flight back home in case of an emergency?
☐ What is your contingency plan if a bad outcome happens?
☐ Have you looked online to find any reviews or stories from previous patients discussing anything negative? Many times, post-surgical infections occur in waves where a

number of patients have surgery around the same time and get the same type of infection.
- Can you afford to travel back to your place of surgery?
- What happens if death occurs? This is a slim but real possibility with all surgery but especially the BBL – 7% death rate out of the country and 1 in 3000 here in the U.S. Is there anyone to sue? How do they get the body home?

If you have read everything so far and you still want to travel for your procedure, we have even more information on the top countries for international medicine to help you make the safest and best decision.

BRAZIL

Brazil is full of beautiful beaches and beautiful women. In 2019, over 1.2 million cosmetic surgery procedures were performed. It's no surprise that people fly to Brazil from all over the world to find some of the best plastic surgeons. Healthcare is a guaranteed right for the citizens of Brazil. In other countries, cosmetic surgery is excluded from free healthcare, but in Brazil it is part of normal medical care because plastic surgeons were able to convince the President and other government leaders that the right to beauty is inherent to the well-being of the people of Brazil. The cosmetic surgery industry in Brazil thrives because the general public has access to plastic surgeons through government-funded medical care. Normally, only a small percentage of a population will entertain plastic surgery, but in Brazil, the government helps lower the cost, and more people take advantage of the benefit.

The higher demand for plastic surgery creates a higher supply of plastic surgeons. They promote and advertise with dramatic before-and-after comparisons to compete for patients and that promotion often catches the attention of American clientele. The best-case scenario always looks amazing, but not every case has a perfect ending. Every year, we hear reports of young women traveling to Brazil for cosmetic procedures and passing away due to surgical complications. While it's true that complications can occur anywhere, you shouldn't take unnecessary risks or ignore warning signs that flash right in front of your face just to save a few hundred dollars.

DOMINICAN REPUBLIC

The Dominican Republic is home to several surgeons who use social media to show off their extreme liposculpting and plastic surgery before and after comparisons. In the DR, there is no regulation that limits the amount of fat removal from the body during a procedure. The more fat that is removed, the more stress is placed on the body. Year after year, tens of thousands of Americans fly to the Dominican Republic for some cosmetic surgical procedure, and every year, dozens of people never come home. In June of 2019, the Dominican Republic Government passed some regulations that require pre-surgical evaluations for all surgical patients.

The horror stories involving patients who traveled to the DR for plastic surgery usually involve a situation where multiple surgeries were performed at one time. An overaggressive surgery plan takes procedures with small risk and adds them together, which causes the risk to increase. If your American surgeon tells you the liposuction you want should be performed in 3 different sessions and you fly to the DR and have it all done in one day, you should expect to have a complication afterwards. What they won't tell you over the phone is that liposuction hurts afterwards. Without routine follow-up, you are left to heal with only the limited amount of pain medication you received overseas and no simple way to get more back home if you need it. You won't be able to get narcotics for your post-surgical pain just by simply asking a random doctor who did not perform your surgery.

MEXICO

In my practice, I see more international follow-up complications from Mexico than any other country. This could be due to how close we are to Mexico, but I also notice that post-op infections are the majority of complications in patients whose surgeries originated in Mexico. Whether deficiency lies with the technique, the cleanliness protocols, or the equipment, the higher risk of infection should not be ignored. Let's face it, if they know you can't afford to do the surgery in the U.S., they also know you can't afford to come back if you have a complication.

Search for "Botched by Baez" on Google or Facebook and see how just one plastic surgeon in Mexico can ruin the lives of so many patients. Earlier this year, dozens of people took advantage of their savings and time off to have plastic surgery in Mexico. In January, two women traveled from San Diego to Tijuana for tummy tucks. Only one returned, and even she developed life-threatening complications that required a two-week recovery in a U.S. hospital. The details she shared with reporters reveal a surgical suite with no monitoring and post-operative recovery that focused more on sedatives than proper care. She developed internal bleeding that caused abdominal compartment syndrome, a complication where the pressure inside the belly is so high, it causes organ failure from poor blood circulation. Her friend died on the operating table. There are dozens of similar stories. The risk of death is real.

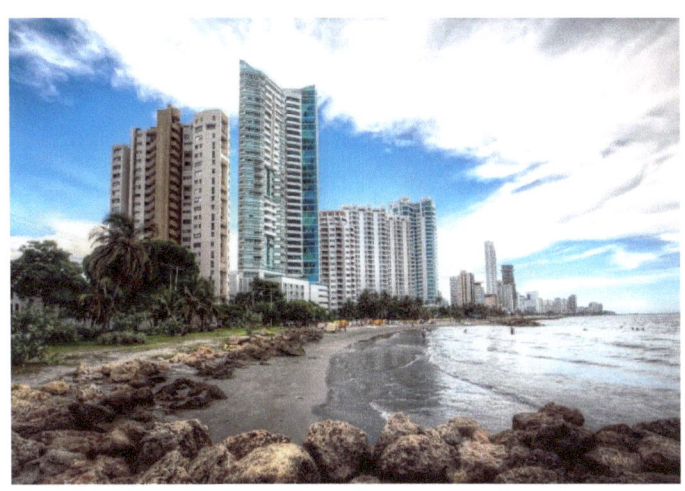

Spirit Airlines now boarding to Colombia!
-Andre Jordan, DDS

Beautiful beaches, beautiful woman, and Pablo Escobar… these are all stereotypes we append to the beautiful South American country of Colombia, which is uniquely located on both the Pacific Ocean and the Caribbean Sea and bookended by Panama and Venezuela. Colombia has quickly risen to the forefront as the most common country that I am asked about with regards to dental tourism. Bogota, Colombia is a four- to five-hour nonstop flight from Houston, Texas. Cali, Bogota, Medellin, and Cartagena are the major cities in Colombia, and they all have dentists that actively advertise to the dental tourists. So, let's dive into why Colombia is one of the countries that we must mention when we talk about dental work 'overseas.

The most common aspect of dental work that motivates people to travel is cosmetic dentistry. Wonder why? Simply put ... SOCIAL MEDIA. The dental industry in Colombia clearly decided to embrace the allure of the country and its reputation for beautiful women to monetize on the worldwide demand for cosmetic dentistry. The formula is simple. First, find a prominent social media personality and give him or her the best dental work possible. Then offer a product that is actually lesser in quality than advertised. Always advertise to a clientele that has champagne taste but beer budget, preferably with a very low dental IQ. Bombard social media with advertising to dominate the market, then reap the benefits.

By dominating the social media landscape with a professional marketing machine, they effectively control the narrative around their products and services. I have personally had patients question my techniques "Do you have to shave down the teeth for veneers?" This question irks me every time. Every patient is different. There are very specific circumstances where shaving down teeth is not required...and in 90% of those instances, it would involve porcelain Lumineers.

Most Colombian veneers take on a bulky, universal white shade, a wholly unattractive appearance. This is due to the fact that they use composite resin, which is the same material used for traditional fillings. In the U.S., composite resin is not placed on top of teeth. Shaving down the teeth is the standard of care in dentistry for cosmetic veneer work. To ask a dentist if the teeth have to be shaved down is analogous to asking if you have to get in a car to drive it. Placing composite material on top of a tooth for the purpose of cosmetics in the typical veneer fashion, as done overseas, also greatly increases the incidence of periodontal disease.

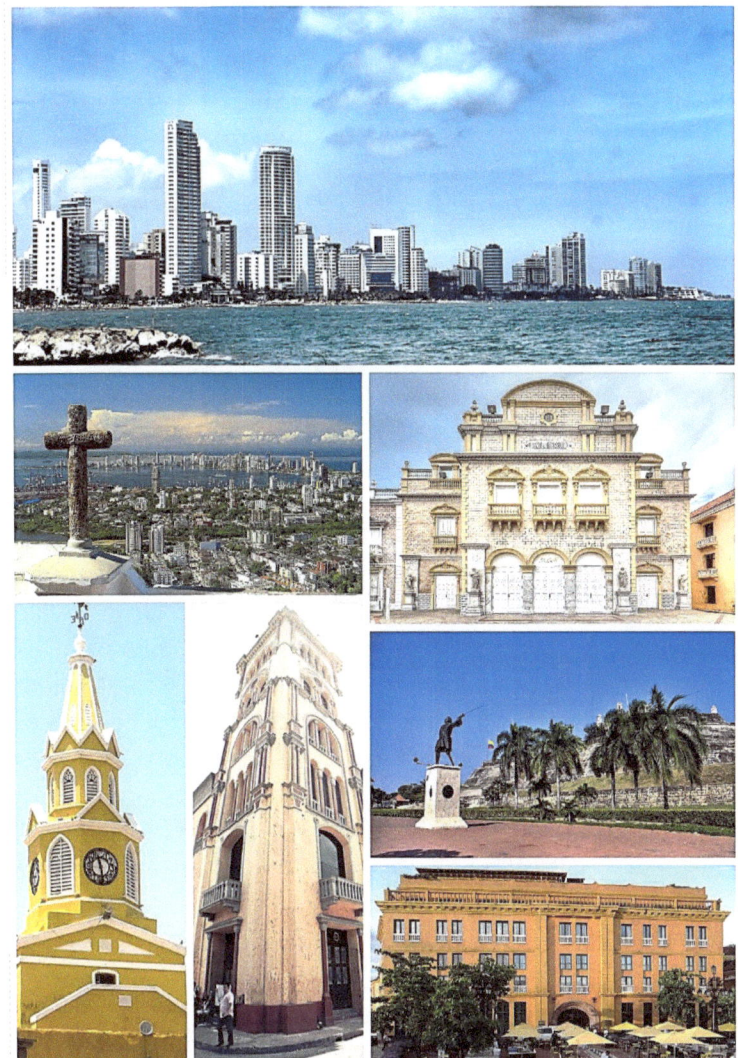

I recently had the pleasure of treating a patient that traveled to Cali, Colombia two weeks earlier where she paid $6000 for veneers, twelve teeth at the top and ten teeth at the bottom. This was an eye-opening experience for me because the patient was very forthcoming with her thoughts on her experience. Typically, people that have traveled out of the country for dental work are not forthcoming with negative experiences due to embarrassment. They usually return to U.S. and search for dentists to fix chipping resin on shoddy veneer work or remove completely failed dental work.

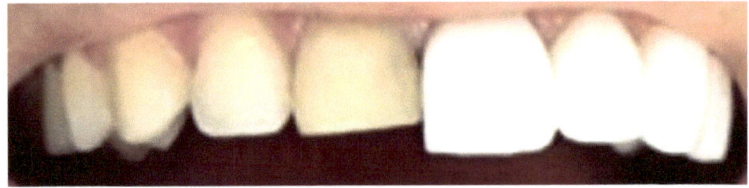

In the case of my patient in question; she stated that she had a feeling that things were not right shortly after the work began. By the time she presented to my office, I noted that the work actually did not look bad at first glance ... sort of a "it looks good from afar but far from good up close". The aesthetics were acceptable; however, every other facet of quality dental work was ignored. What I saw indicated that the work was performed by a clinician who either legitimately lacked dental knowledge or rushed the work. The lingual side (the back side) of the teeth demonstrated a lack of adherence to the principles of jaw movement and occlusion...in lay terms...the patient could not close her mouth all the way. As such, she could not eat without pain in her teeth or jaw. The veneer material was placed without regard to her anatomy, causing sores to develop on her tongue due to an improper rest position. Overall, she was living in misery.

Let's talk about the quality of the composite resins. In America we utilize the composite resin for fillings or temporary material. In the locations that these veneers are placed, namely the front teeth; they are primarily exposed to cutting and shearing forces that are tangential in direction. Composite resin ranks very low in its ability to withstand all of those elements. Due to the properties of composite resin, it is completely forbidden in patients that grind their teeth.

How does Colombia compare to America in terms of the dental education and practical experience acquired in dental school? The road to becoming a dentist in Colombia is roughly 4 years shorter than in America. Honestly, it functions more akin to a trade school. Dental school in Colombia is comprised of a 5-year curriculum, a year longer than the American regimen of 4 years; however, dental school in Colombia begins immediately after high school, provided the students pass a career placement exam. In America, admission to dental school is dependent upon demonstrating a comprehension of collegiate level sciences and other relevant prerequisites. These requirements are absent in the Colombian process, and if the public were aware, it should be a glaring red flag. Given the lower bar of entry into Dental school in Colombia, it should be no surprise that the dental industry in Colombia is saturated. The very high number of dentists in Colombia compete against each other so much, many are unemployed.

The savvy traveler would also ask if traveling to Colombia is safe before researching Colombian cosmetic dentists. Colombia has a historical link to crime that is unrivaled by any other country. From the long running drug empire as romanticized by Scarface and Pablo Escobar to the guerillas of the Marxist rebel group FARC (Fuerza Alternativa Revolucionaria del Comun). The FARC, notorious for kidnappings, guerilla warfare, and terrorism, currently have a 'truce' with the Colombian government. The more prevalent risk of danger in Colombia would lie with the run-of-the-mill street crime that you might encounter almost anywhere. If you do decide to travel to Colombia, be cautious and protect yourself with the typical defensive precautions you would use as a tourist in any country.

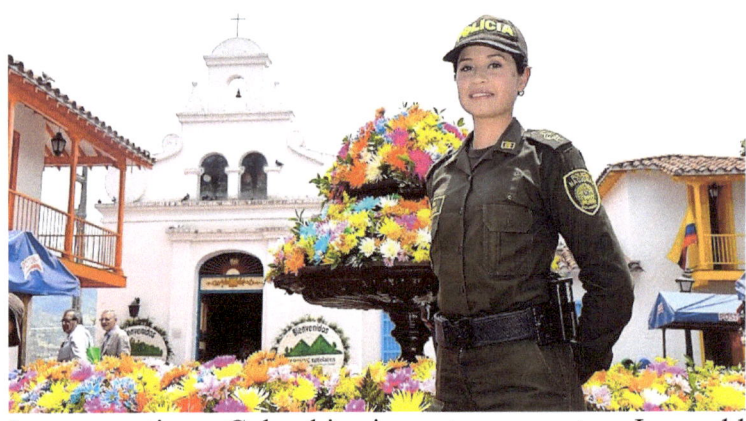

In summation, Colombia is not a country I would recommend traveling to for advanced dental work or cosmetic dental procedures. While Colombia is a highly developed nation with a large population of dentists, their baseline training lacks the fundamentals that would inspire confidence in advanced work. Furthermore, there is no governing body that will uphold your patient rights as a non-citizen. I would not hesitate to allow a Colombian trained dentist to perform routine dental care; however, the cost of travel and lost time due to distance negates any financial savings incentive. The exchange rate at time of print between the U.S. Dollar and the Colombian Peso is 1 to 3,805, which accounts for a large portion of the patient savings for high-cost procedures. The lopsided exchange rate benefits the Colombian dentist who pays rent and purchases materials with Pesos but is paid in U.S. dollars.

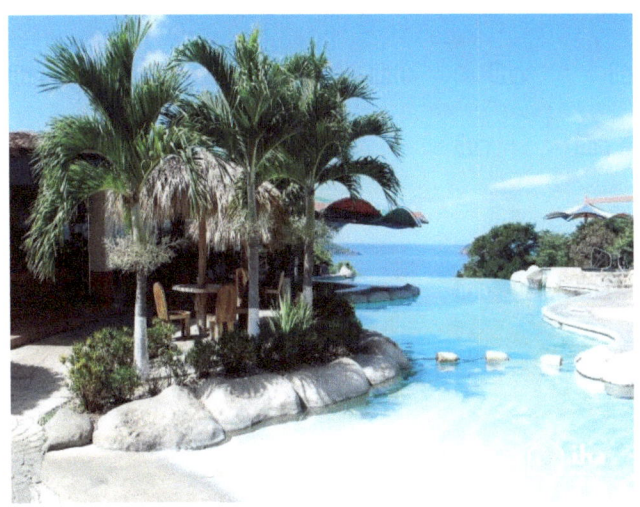

Costa Rica – Pura Vida!

-Andre Jordan, DDS

Costa Rica is a beautiful country in Central America bookended by the Isthmus of Panama and Nicaragua. It is a country that I have made several trips to and have been astounded with how much natural beauty exists there. I have always maintained the opinion that of all the countries I have visited, Costa Rica is one country where I would not have as many reservations about having my dental work performed. Travel to Costa Rica is a two-and-a-half to three-hour flight from Miami or Houston, so it ranks as one of the more accessible destinations for dental tourism. Due to this close proximity, a good number of American ex-patriates who reside in Costa Rica, which means that there is a good chance that you may find a dentist that actually attended dental school or a post-graduate program in the United States. But, if you happen to schedule with a local dentist, let's talk about the requirements for becoming a dentist in Costa Rica versus the United States.

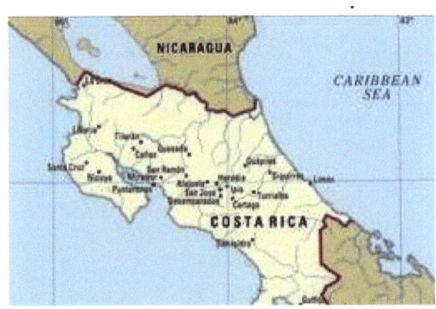

Costa Rica, unlike the United States, allows dental candidates to enter dental school without obtaining any collegiate level prerequisite education. The caveat lies in that the Costa Rican dental school curriculum is six years long, compared to four years in the United States. The two-year difference in the Costa Rican dental education system can be rationalized out in that the two years added could be the equivalent of any 'knowledge' lost from not having the American standard of prerequisite courses. Dentists in Costa Rica demonstrate a command of the dental craft that has built confidence in the industry. Costa Rica ranks as one of the top countries that I actually do recommend to people that ask me about dental tourism…if they are insistent upon leaving the United States for treatment. As of June 2021, there are five dental programs in Costa Rica, which is not a surprising number given the size of the country. Three of the dental programs are located in the heart of the country where the capital of San Jose lies. Costa Rica has a universal healthcare system with standardized government reimbursement that reduces the bottom-line income of Costa Rican dentists; therefore, it was wise for the Costa Rican industry to invest in dental and medical tourism. What are the cost differences exactly?

In my personal visits to Costa Rica, I can tell you that any financial savings that would be realized are based in the exchange rate. At time of print, one U.S. Dollar was worth 616 Costa Rican Colón. The exchange rate would be responsible for driving the material costs down. This is an important talking point as we begin to look at specific dental procedures, namely, implants. Implant placement is about the only dental procedure I would endorse when looking for dental treatment in Costa Rica. The exchange rate and the cost of travel does not equate to any financial savings for any other dental treatment. Yes, the deal hunters will say that the overall out-of-pocket cost may still be lower by a few hundred dollars but is it worth the "what ifs?". What if the dental work fails, what if there are complications, what if the treatment requires multiple visits? At that point, the financial savings begins to be negated by the cost of not having peace of mind.

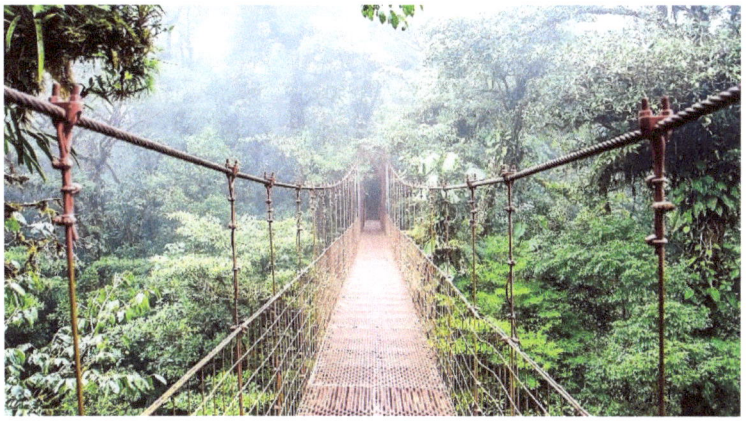

Unlike most countries we discuss in the book, Costa Rica has a trustworthy dental governing body that regulates and administers the practice of dentistry akin to various United States dental boards. With regards to safety in Costa Rica, having travelled there several times, I have never felt any more or any less safe than in the United States. Obviously, the capital city of San Jose presents with the safety challenges of any metropolitan area in the world. When you venture out to the resort areas of Jaco, Herradura, and Guanacaste, you may encounter dangers that are more natural than man-made.

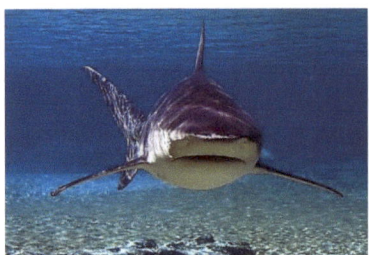 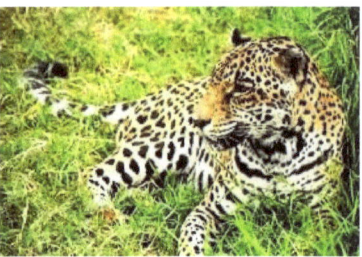

Costa Rica is a cornucopia of wild beauty courtesy of mother nature. On excursions in the jungle and forays to the beach you can encounter vanilla and aloe vera growing wild, toucans and parrots flying by, sloths and spider monkeys literally hanging in the forest, and stingrays and dolphins in their natural habitats. It truly is a wonderous sight, but the flip side to that beauty are the natural predators that lurk behind it. Bull Sharks and Tiger Sharks are native to the coastal waters. Jaguars stalk the jungle peaks, while crocodiles and caimans lurk in the waterways in between. Venomous spiders and scorpions dot the jungle floor as well as the crevices of Airbnb rentals.

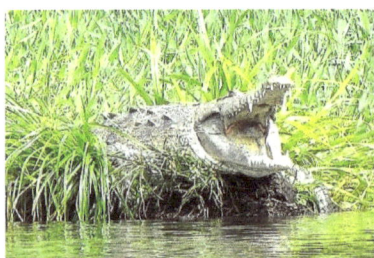 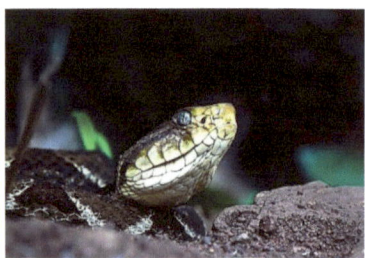

Costa Rica is also home to one of the deadliest snakes in the Americas, the fer-de-lance, a highly venomous asper of the pit viper family. The fer-de-lance causes the most snakebite-related deaths in Central America, so you don't want to meet one up close. I personally have seen half of the predators listed; as such I can say don't venture too far off the beaten path without a guide if you haven't at least watched your fair share of National Geographic.

In summation, I like Costa Rica. I believe that when the exchange rate is favorable, it can bring down the cost of labor and materials below that of the United States, so it's worth consideration for implant treatment. The exchange rate is not favorable enough to save money on routine dental work and less expensive procedures. The main consideration is that if you do embark on dental treatment in Costa Rica, factor in the need for follow-up dental visits in the U.S. along with your travel costs.

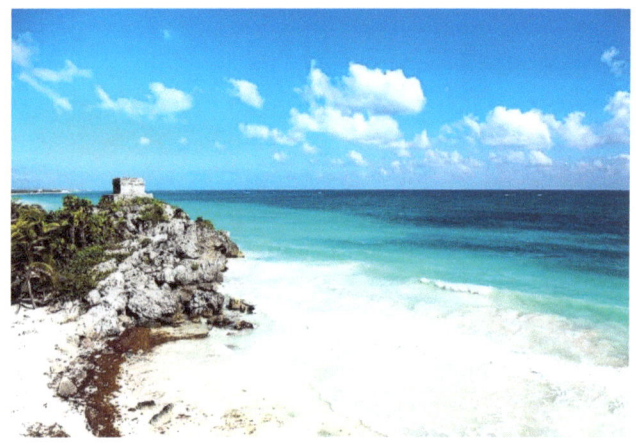

Bienvenidos a Mexico!

-Andre Jordan, DDS

After a decade of practicing dentistry in Texas, I have A LOT of exposure to Mexican sourced dental work. My anecdotal experiences range from follow ups on excellent dental work to correcting the absolute worst dental work that I have ever seen. Our proximity to Mexico, less than a two-hour flight to Cancun beaches from Houston, has also created another dental tourist option for patients looking to save a few bucks. I personally know several people that have traveled to Mexico for dental work. Along the Texas border cities of McAllen, Brownsville, Laredo, and El Paso you will find large outposts of dental tourism. There are also many Mexican trained general dentists that have filtered into the ancillary industries of dentistry. I'm talking about dental labs, dental assisting, and dental education. Let's dive into the dental industry of our next-door neighbor to the south!

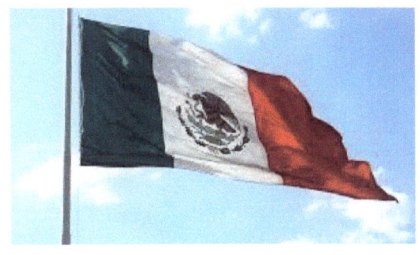

What does it take to become a dentist in Mexico? Unfortunately, not much. Training to become a dentist in Mexico rivals that of a barber college in the United States. Specifically, this means that there is a deficit of approximately four to six years of formal education! The other blaring issue that exists is that there is no formal governing body to supervise the practice of dentistry in Mexico. Translation…it's the wild west. In the United States, dental enforcement is carried out by each state's respective dental board and any dentist will get a chill that runs down their spine at the mere mention of a state dental board visit. Imagine a world where your trusted, or not-so-trusted, clinician is the final word, with no concern for oversight, no risk of reprimand, and no fear of governance. There is virtually no way to research a dentist's credentials or reputation in Mexico. Without an established and trustworthy system of maintaining standards of practice, the only real method of vetting a dentist in Mexico is via referrals. The other issue that raises more concern than the credentials of the dentists in Mexico is the uncertainty of the origin or type of materials.

I have a family friend who had been going to Mexico with his family for all of their dental work. One day, he contacted me from McAllen, TX with great concern in his voice. He sent me a pic of his face and his upper lip was swollen three times normal size after recent dental work. I was as concerned as he was. I could not help him much because we [he and I] could not tell what material was used…or whether it was sanctioned or even expired. Fortunately, his lip returned to normal after 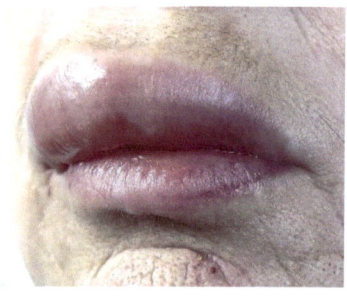 a few days. I can personally attest to the alien origin of some of the materials used. In my office, I have seen and removed some Mexican dental work, and I couldn't decipher what type of metal it was or what method of installation was utilized. For an American trained dentist – this is more than eyebrow raising. This story underscores the most troublesome issue with dental tourism in Mexico. The materials, equipment, or sterilization protocols are not regulated either. You have even less of a forum to vet the cleanliness of any dental office that you may visit in Mexico than you do to vet the actual dentist.

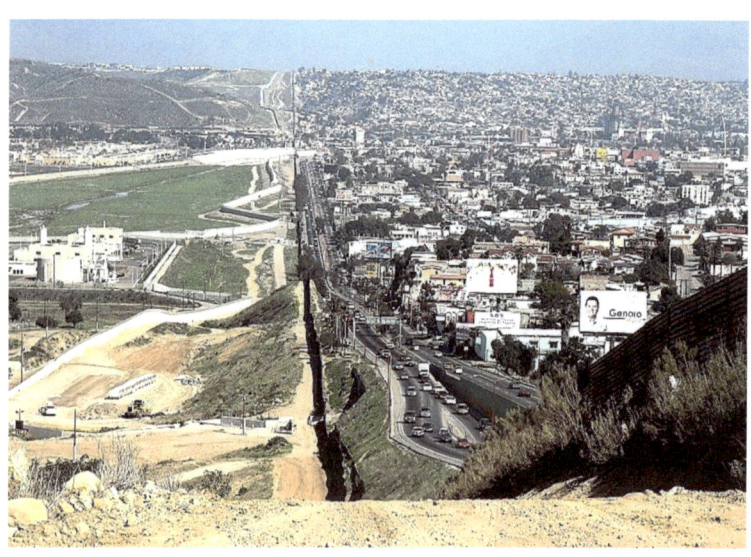

The final concern of Mexico based dental tourism is the inherent danger of traveling to Mexico. Of course, there are certain areas that are safer than others, however, across the board Mexico is fraught with violence. In certain regions, the Mexican cartel is waging war against the police and government. You have to exercise extreme caution if you travel to traditionally non-tourist areas of Mexico.

My honest opinion is that Mexican dental work is only worthwhile if you have close friends or relatives in Mexico that can properly vet the clinician that you are trying to see. The implant systems are foreign sourced at best, and the risk of catastrophic failure is a chance that you may not want to take. If you have already visited Mexico for dental work and escaped any negative effects, you have traversed a gauntlet that would frighten away most patients with a dash of Kokura's Luck. Kokura's Luck refers to surviving a situation of imminent danger and not ever being aware of it. I don't know of any dental procedure that I can recommend going to Mexico for that justifies the inherent health and mortality risk.

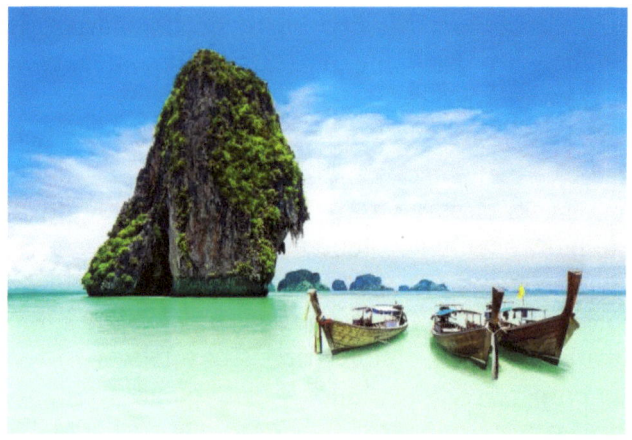

Phuket! Let's go to Thailand!
-Andre Jordan, DDS

Thailand is one of my favorite countries that I have had the pleasure of visiting. Thailand has emerged as a new leading destination for dental tourism in the last five to ten years. It is also one of the countries that I feel more confident in endorsing dental tourism if one must embark upon that journey. Let's establish why Thailand is rising in such popularity for dental work.

As with any other country, the appeal for dental tourism has to be rooted in the economics of the dental work. As with many other countries, the cost of work is directly tied to the exchange rate. At print, the Thai Bhat is worth 0.03 USD, which by itself makes Thailand and extremely popular tourist destination. The last time I was in Thailand (Bangkok and Phuket), I ate three good meals a day for about $10 to $20 USD. I stayed in a suite at the hotel Le Bua which was featured in 'The Hangover Part II' for about $120 USD per night! I recommend visiting Thailand on the strength of the exchange rate alone. As opposed to other popular Asian tourist locales, Thailand – Bangkok in particular…is not the cleanest of cities. Hong Kong, Tokyo, and Singapore all are spotless by comparison. Don't let this necessarily deter you from certain dental procedures there. Let's discover why.

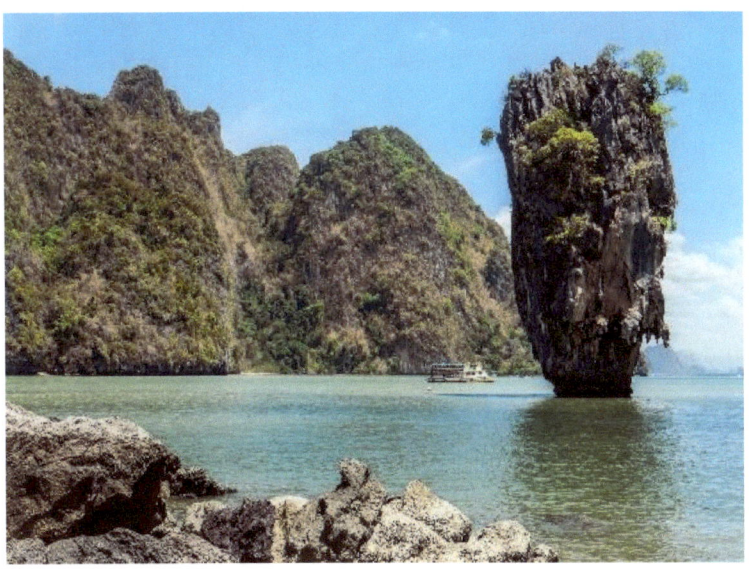

What does it take to become a dentist in Thailand? Thailand, like most countries featured in this book, does not require formal collegiate level education prior to enrolling in dental school. The dental school curriculum consists of six years of education, which is two years short in comparison to the United States when you combine the four-year collegiate degree requirement with a four-year dental program. The pivotal factor that leads me to feel more comfortable with dental work in Thailand is the fact that after the six-year dental school program to lead to the DDS degree, every dentist is then required to work in the public dental system for an additional three years. Having personally practiced in public health dentistry – I can attest strongly to the value of the experience a clinician can receive from practicing in public health.

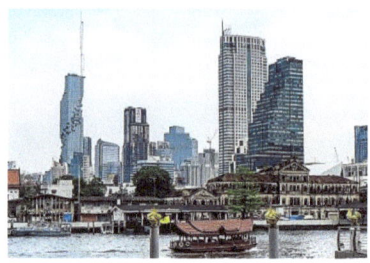 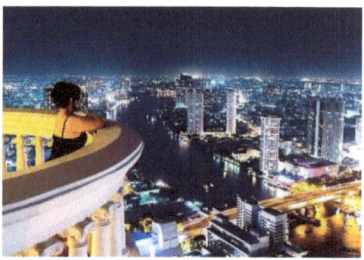

Now we turn our attention toward the drawbacks of traveling to Thailand for dental work. The universal downside to all dental tourism is the lack of any type of practical guarantee or ability to follow up with your treating doctor. Both sides understand that the cost of flying back prevents most tourism patients from acting on any promise of free follow-up. Of the countries we cover, Thailand has the longest distance and travel time, so the universal downside is even more prominent. If you are reading this book and reside in the United States of America, a trip to Thailand is a very far jaunt. As of June 2021, there are zero nonstop flights from the United States to Thailand, and no airlines have any immediate plans for one. From America you will have to transit another large Asian hub or go via Europe or the Middle East. This creates a cumulative travel time of 18 hours at best, and well over 24 hours on some itineraries. You might be able to plan a ten- or fourteen-day trip for your initial dental work, which provides time to catch any short-term complications. Unfortunately, midterm to long-term complications that may arise will almost certainly occur after you have departed Southeast Asia.

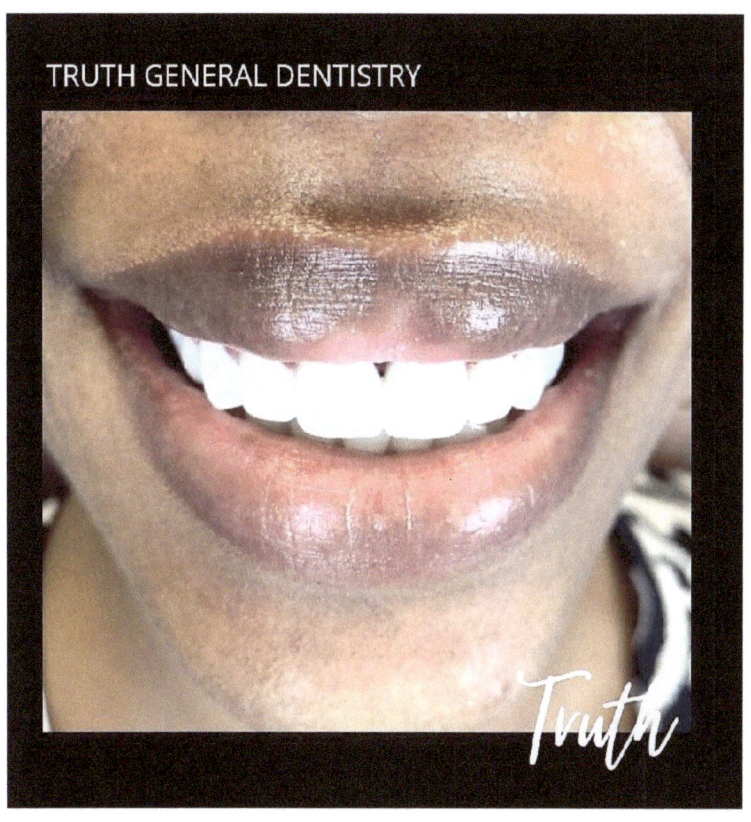

One final note - you have to remember that at the end of every tooth is one heart, two lungs, two kidneys etc. We as dental clinicians – we do not merely treat teeth – we treat people with teeth. Once you grasp the fundamental connection that the actions you take with your mouth affects the health of your entire body; you will become more discerning about who performs your dental care – here and abroad.

About the Authors

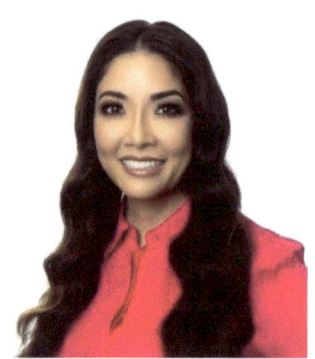

Erika Sato, MD is certified by both the American Board of Plastic Surgery and the American Board of Surgery, Dr. Erika Sato specializes in cosmetic surgery of the face, breast, and body. She performs the latest treatments in cosmetic surgery as well as nonsurgical rejuvenation. Dr. Sato is committed to providing excellence in care, while treating every patient like family.

A Missouri native, Dr. Sato was drawn to the field of plastic surgery when she was diagnosed with Binder's Syndrome as a child. Binder's syndrome is a rare congenital malformation resulting in undergrowth of the central face and may include elements of the nose and upper jaw. She underwent rhinoplasty surgery as a teenager utilizing cartilage from her right ear to reconstruct her nose. At just 15 years old she experienced how life changing plastic surgery can be and knew that she wanted to be a plastic surgeon, so that someday she could impact others' lives in a similar manor.

After graduating from the Honors College at the University of Missouri – Columbia with a Bachelor of Science in Biology with a Pre-Med emphasis, Dr. Sato went on to finish medical school at the University of Missouri – Columbia School of Medicine. She then completed her general surgery residency at The University of Texas Health Science Center at Houston in the world-renowned Texas Medical Center followed by a rigorous fellowship in Plastic and Reconstructive Surgery at the same institution.

In 2015, Dr. Sato was featured as a main cast member on Bravo's reality TV show *Married to Medicine Houston*. Dr. Sato has won dozens of awards, including Top Doctors 2020 by Houstonia Magazine, RealSelf 100 & 500 Hall of Fame Distinguished Inductee, Top 100 by RealSelf 2017, Texas Monthly's Super Doctors: Rising Stars 2017, 2019 & 2020, and Houston Top Doctor by H Texas Magazine 2016 – 2019.

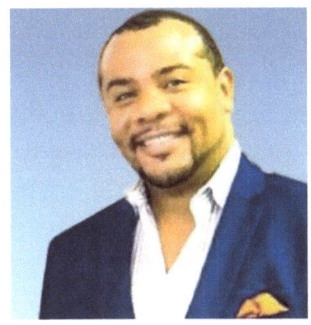

Dr. Andre Jordan is a native Houstonian and proud of it. Dr. Jordan graduated from the DeBakey High School for Health Professions and earned a Bachelor of Science Degree in Psychology with a minor in Chemistry from Xavier University of New Orleans, Louisiana.

Dr. Jordan attended Meharry Medical College School of Dentistry of Nashville, Tennessee, where he earned his Doctorate of Dental Surgery in 2011. He has worked in various aspects of dentistry while building a strong following in the community. He is an active member of Kappa Alpha Psi Fraternity Incorporated as well as various dental organizations. Dr. Jordan believes that the dental landscape of the Houston area has become littered with corporate entities that place profit over the care of the patient, and his motto is to "Dare to Disrupt".

In 2015, he founded Truth General Dentistry, a fresh take on modern dentistry focused on providing the highest quality dental care with refreshing honesty and transparency.

Final Thoughts

Everyone always says you only live once when they want to justify crazy behavior, but nobody wants to be the one to fly home in a bag under the plane instead of inside the main cabin. All surgery comes with risk, but that doesn't mean that the risk is equal everywhere. International travel is sexy and alluring, so it's easy to see why patients get caught up in the moment. Just remember that advertising is designed to show you what they want you to see while hiding what they want to keep hidden. Do your research and use the info in this book to guide you to a safe and sound decision. Enjoy your Hot Girl Summer body all year long, just don't get Botched!

Follow us on IG:

@dr.erikasato, @dredds1911, @er_doctor_o

Read more of our books available at
http://thebp.site/267048
http://thebp.site/291063